Suélem Lavorato de Oliveira
Rafael Haddad Manfio
Isabela Bazzo Costa

Standardisation of Semen Collection in Three Snake Species

Suélem Lavorato de Oliveira
Rafael Haddad Manfio
Isabela Bazzo Costa

Standardisation of Semen Collection in Three Snake Species

ScienciaScripts

Imprint

Any brand names and product names mentioned in this book are subject to trademark, brand or patent protection and are trademarks or registered trademarks of their respective holders. The use of brand names, product names, common names, trade names, product descriptions etc. even without a particular marking in this work is in no way to be construed to mean that such names may be regarded as unrestricted in respect of trademark and brand protection legislation and could thus be used by anyone.

Cover image: www.ingimage.com

This book is a translation from the original published under ISBN 978-613-9-72657-8.

Publisher:
Sciencia Scripts
is a trademark of
Dodo Books Indian Ocean Ltd. and OmniScriptum S.R.L publishing group

120 High Road, East Finchley, London, N2 9ED, United Kingdom
Str. Armeneasca 28/1, office 1, Chisinau MD-2012, Republic of Moldova, Europe
Printed at: see last page
ISBN: 978-620-7-90320-7

SUMMARY

The application of reproductive biotechnologies to wild animals has increased in recent years. In the case of reptiles, the reasons for this are the restriction of animal imports, a reduction in the introduction of diseases, an increase in the number of endangered species, making it possible to exchange genetic material, reducing costs, rapid population growth, promoting gamete and/or embryo banking, among others. The aim of this work was to standardise semen collection from snake species from different families, Epicrates crassus, Python regius and *Crotalus durissus terrificus. The* samples were collected at IPEVS - Instituto de Pesquisa em Vida Selvagem e Meio Ambiente, using the technique described by Mengden (1980), which consists of ventral massage of the final third of the animal's body and the ejaculate is collected with a syringe. The collection proved satisfactory for *C. durissus*, thus collecting viable sperm, while for *E. crassus* and *P. regius the collection was* not effective because the sperm were immobile. This may be related to the diet of these two species, which are constrictors with more developed muscles, making massage difficult.

Keywords: Reptiles. Reproduction. Biotechnology. Males.

SUMMARY

CHAPTER 1

INTRODUCTION

Snakes belong to the Kingdom Animalia, Class Reptilia, Order Squamata and Suborder Serpentes. They originated in the Cretaceous period, but developed in the Cenozoic, and appear to be part of a group of lizards (GREGO, 2014; ANDRADE; 2002).

They are found in various regions of the planet, from tropical forests to deserts, oceans and even temperate zones, but the tropical and temperate regions are where they occur most frequently, which is explained by the fact that they are ectothermic beings, so they depend on external temperature to maintain their physiological characteristics. The environments they occupy are aquatic, arboreal, terrestrial and fossorial (GREGO, 2014; ANDRADE, 2002; ZACARIOTTI, 2008).

The reproductive anatomy of male snakes is made up of two asymmetrically arranged testes, the right one being larger and more cranial than the left. They are ovoid, elongated and cylindrical masses, located intra-abdominally, cranially to the kidneys. They are connected to the base of the hemipenis, the copulatory organ, by the ductus deferens (PIZZATO, 2006a; MATAYOSHI, 2011; ALMEIDA-SANTOS, 2014; ZACARIOTTI, 2004; ZACARIOTTI, 2008).

Sexual dimorphism may be present in some snake species, as exemplified by the relationship between body dimensions (PIZZATTO, 2006a), the number and shape of scales, the position and size of glands or organs, and colouration (ZACARIOTTI, 2008).

The male's reproductive cycle is basically made up of energy acquisition, spermatogenesis, production of secondary sexual characteristics, search for copulations, dance combat, courtship and copulations (ZACARIOTTI, 2008). In them, energy is acquired by feeding and thus storing abdominal fat during the summer (SUEIRO, 2013).

Today, with the destruction of habitats, wild animals are becoming extinct. As a result, reproduction techniques are essential to enable the exchange of genetic material, allow the reproduction of animals with physical limitations, enable rapid population growth, manage the social ratio, determine the offspring and promote the formation of gamete banks. The aim of this study was to standardise the collection of semen from three different snake species: Epicrates crassus from the Boidae family, Python regius from the Pitonidae family and Crotalus durissus terrificus from the Viperidae family.

CHAPTER 2

LITERATURE REVIEW

2.1. Snake biology

2.1.1 Biology of Epicrates crassus

Table 1: Scientific classification of Epicrates crassus (Adapted from GREGO, 2014);

SCIENTIFIC CLASSIFICATION	
Kingdom	Animalia
Class	Reptilia
Order	Squamata
Suborder	Snakes
Family	Boidae
Gender	*Epicrates*
Species	*Usicrates crassus*
Common name	Salamanta or Cerrado Rainbow boa

The Epicrates complex is found in all Neotropical regions, occurring in portions of South and Central America (Figure 5). Epicrates crassus are found in open formations in Brazil, Bolivia and Argentina (PASSOS, 2008). With nocturnal and diurnal habits, they are usually observed in terrestrial or arboreal environments (GARCIA, 2012, CHARLES, 2007).

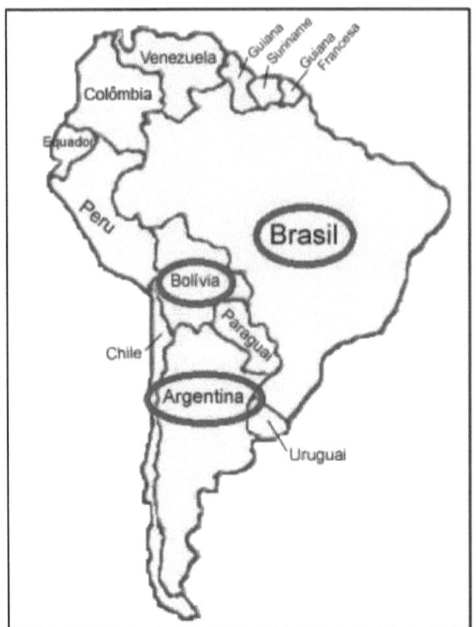

Figure 1: Geographical distribution of *Epicrates crassus* (regions outlined in red) (Public domain image modified);

They range in colour from brown to red, the back is usually reddish-brown and shiny, the side is greyish, with several circular black spots distributed mainly on the back and sides, and can also be called furta-coloured, while the belly is white and without spots. The head is quite distinct from the neck, with the rostral part being wider than it is high, and the head also has longitudinal dark lines running from the eyes and nostrils. The labial scales have fossae, resembling folds. The eyes have a black iris with a vertical pupil. Both males and females can measure approximately 2 metres in length (Figure 6) (FRAGA, 2013; CARVALHO, 2007; CHARLES, 2007).

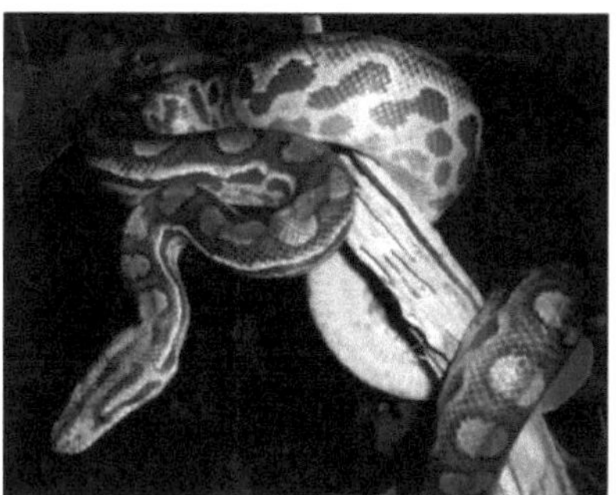

Figure 2: Epicrates crassus (Salamanta) (Public domain image);

They have aglyph teeth, i.e. they don't have venom-inoculating teeth. They feed on small mammals such as mice, birds, embryonated eggs and lizards (SCARTOZZONI, 2004; PASSOS, 2008). They are viviparous snakes, with vitellogenesis occurring in the autumn and winter, so the birth of the young is in the rainy season, spring and summer (GARCIA, 2012; PRADO, 2006).

2.1.2 Biology of Python regius

Table 2: Scientific classification of Python regius (Adapted from GREGO, 2014);

SCIENTIFIC CLASSIFICATION	
Kingdom	Animalia
Class	Reptilia
Order	Squamata
Suborder	Snakes
Family	Pitonidae
Gender	*Python*
Species	*Sython regius*
Common name	Ball python or Royal python

Python regius are found in several African countries such as Nigeria, Uganda, Sudan and others (Figure 7). Their habits are nocturnal and they have a terrestrial habitat, which is why they are found in dry pastures, open forests, farmland, abandoned burrows and among dry leaves (GREGO, 2014; PRADO, 2006).

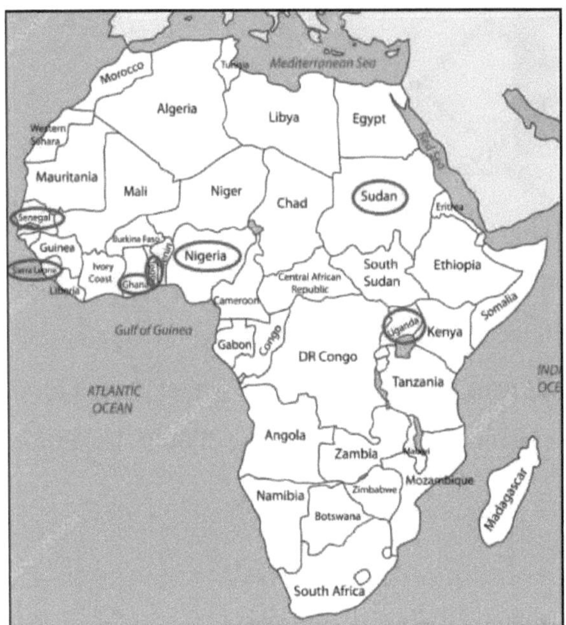

Figure 3: Geographical distribution of Python regius (regions outlined in red) (Public domain image modified);

When they are born, they measure between 25 and 43 cm. Their adult length can reach 1.5 metres, but there have been reports of animals up to 1.83 metres, but females are usually larger than males. Its head is larger than its neck and its body has brown spots interspersed with light spots. It may also have yellowish spots on its nostrils and eyes and its belly is white (Figure 8) (GRAF, 2011). When it feels threatened, it curls up on its own body in the shape of a ball, hence the common name "ball python" (IRIZARRY, 2016).

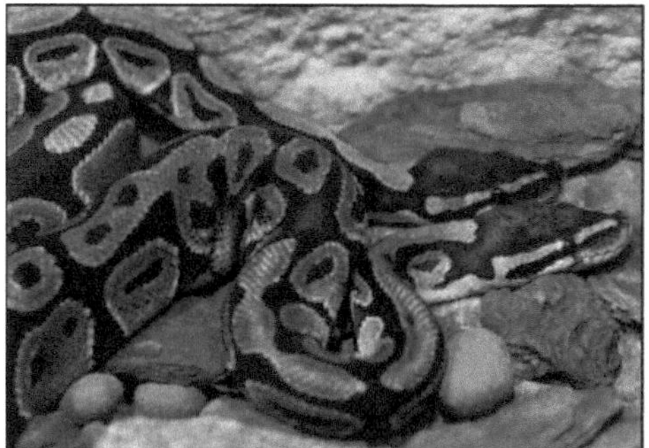

Figure 4: Python regius (Ball python) (Public domain image);

Their teeth, like those of the Salamantas, are aglyphous and do not have venom-inoculating teeth. Birds and small rodents are part of their diet. They are oviparous snakes, with embryonic development inside the egg. They are late-blooming animals, reaching sexual maturity at the age of 5 and females reproduce every 2-3 years. After mating, an average of 10 eggs are laid in a protected place, where the mother surrounds the eggs with her body and stays with them most of the time, alert to intruders and the needs of her future offspring. The incubation period lasts a maximum of 80 days (GREGO, 2014).

2.1.3 Biology of Crotalus durissus terrificus

Table 3: Scientific classification of Crotalus durissus terrificus (Adapted from GREGO, 2014);

SCIENTIFIC CLASSIFICATION	
Kingdom	Animalia
Class	Reptilia
Order	Squamata
Suborder	Snakes
Family	Viperidae
Gender	*Crotalus*
Species	*Crotalus durissus tencficus*
Common name	Rattlesnake

Crotalus durissus terrificus is found almost everywhere in Brazil, with the exception of most of the northern region, but is mainly found in the Cerrado (Figure 9). It has a terrestrial habit and lives in open fields and dry, rocky regions, and is active at night, but can be found active during twilight (GREGO, 2014; COSTA, 2008).

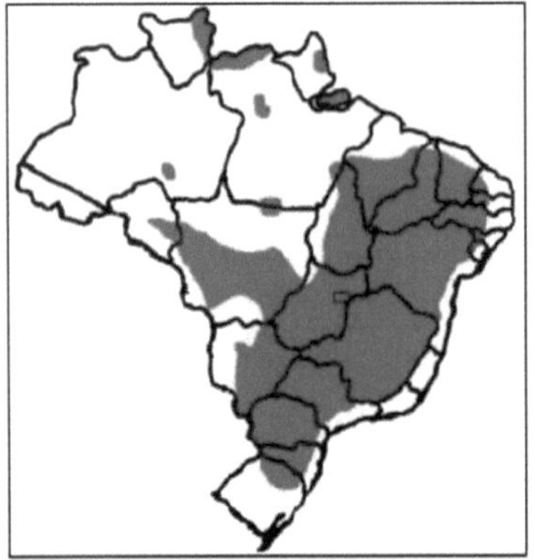

Figure 5: Geographical distribution of Crotallus durissus terrificus (Source: Instituto Butantan);

Its main characteristic is the presence of a rattle, found on the tip of its tail, which produces sound. It is yellowish-brown in colour, with lighter diamond-shaped designs on its back and sides (GREGO, 2014). It has a structure called the loreal fossa, which has the function of thermoregulation and is found on the head between the eyes and the nostril. Its length is approximately 1.20 metres (Figure 10) (FRAGA, 2013).

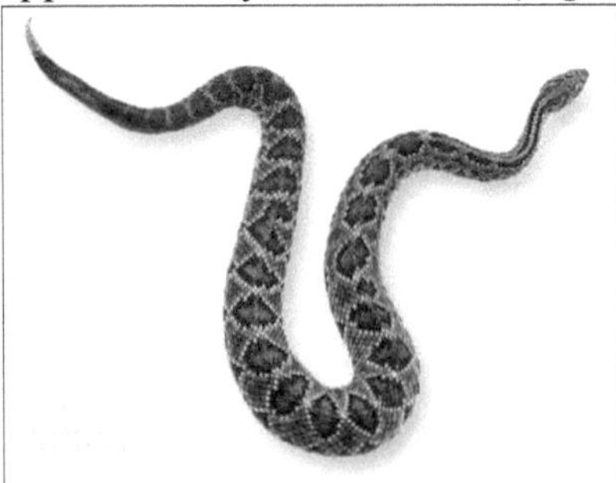

Figure 6: Crotalus durissus terrificus (Rattlesnake) (Public domain image);

They have solenoglyphic teeth, i.e. two venom-inoculating teeth.

Their basic diet consists of small mammals such as rodents. They are viviparous snakes where the females have a reproductive cycle between the end of the dry season and the beginning of the rainy season, from August to November, while the males reproduce throughout the year. Gestation lasts an average of 4 months and around 25 offspring are born in rainy seasons such as summer (GREGO, 2014).

2.2   Reproductive anatomy

In both sexes, the reproductive organs are paired and asymmetrical, with the right usually being more cranial and larger than the left (Figure 11) (MATAYOSHI, 2011; ALMEIDA-SANTOS, 2014). They are ovoid, elongated, cylindrical and located intra-abdominally in the coelomic cavity between the gallbladder, spleen, pancreas, which makes up the pancreatic triad, and the kidneys. They are made up of seminiferous tubules, interstitial cells and blood vessels, surrounded by connective tissue and tunica propria.

(ZACARIOTTI, 2004; PIZZATO, 2006a; ZACARIOTTI, 2008; ALMEIDA-SANTOS, 2014; MATAYOSHI, 2011).

Communication between the testicles and the cloaca is provided by the vas deferens, which morphologically are coiled in active males and smooth in immature ones, ending in the genital papillae, near the base of the penis, which are common pathways between the genital and urinary tract, where the spermatic groove is located, as reptiles do not have a penile urethra (MATAYOSHI, 2011; ZACARIOTTI, 2008).

The efferent ducts are distributed along the entire length of the testicles and are orientated towards the epididymis, which does not differentiate into head, body and tail, as in mammals, but is closely linked to the testicles

(ALMEIDA-SANTOS, 2005). The ampulla is located in the final third of the ductus deferens. In snakes, it has the function of storing sperm, but there have been few studies when compared to mammals, which have the function of maturing, nourishing, storing and phagocytosing sperm (ALMEIDA-SANTOS, 2014).

In squamates, the copulatory organ is a pair, called hemipenis, which are located inside the tail when copulation is not taking place (ZACARIOTTI, 2008). In all snakes, only one of the hemipenis is introduced during copulation (ZACARIOTTI, 2010). It is a spongy organ, which fills with blood and lymph at the moment of erection, and also has some differentiations such as spines and other macro- and micro-ornamentation (ANDRADE, 2002). In rattlesnakes, the hemipenis is bilobed and with

structures for attachment at the moment of copulation, such as hooks and papillae (ZACARIOTTI, 2004).

As external sexual dimorphism in snakes is difficult, sexing is done by placing a blunt, metallic, lubricated probe in the cloaca, where in males it is inserted up to 12 subcaudal scales and in females four scales (GREGO, 2014). However, in some species the tail can be seen to be longer in males than in females (PIZZATO, 2006a).

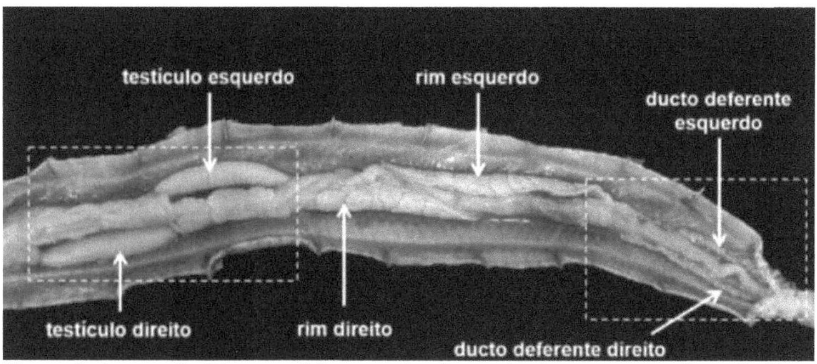

Figure 7: Anatomical layout of the reproductive and urinary organs of a male Xenodon sp. (Source: ALMEIDA-SANTOS, 2014).

1.1.1. Ultrasound assessment

Ultrasound is a non-invasive diagnostic method that provides numerous assessments of the same individual without euthanising them. In general, the most commonly used equipment are linear transducers with frequencies of 5.0 to 7.5 MHz and 7.5 to 10 MHz, as described by MATAYOSHI (2012), respectively, but this can vary according to the size of the patient.

To carry out the examination, the animal needs to be physically restrained. Sedation or anaesthesia is rarely used, especially in very active or aggressive animals. The patient is then positioned in the ventral or sternal decubitus position, as the acoustic window is through the lateral wall or ventral surface of the middle third at the end of the coelomatic cavity. For the best image definition, the gel should be applied 5 to 30 minutes before the examination, as it penetrates the scales and reduces the air interface. Another technique used is immersing the animal in warm water (MATAYOSHI, 2011).

During the examination, the reference point is the gallbladder, located in the middle third of the coelomic cavity, as the reproductive organs are detected caudally to it. For males, the ultrasound scan is important because it assesses reproductive conditions, with information on the size and development of the testicles. When they are inactive, they are hardly observed, but during the reproductive period the parenchyma is granular and of medium echogenicity, forming a homogeneous and hypoechogenic image (GARCIA, 2015; MATAYOSHI, 2011). In the case of females, the parenchyma is hyperechoic, but with initial follicles that are anechoic and then hyperechoic (ALMEIDA, 2010).

1.2. Reproductive Biology

As they are ectothermic animals, they are vulnerable to the environment, so with the variation in body temperature there is a change in the animal's ecophysiological condition. The changes that most affect reptiles are environmental temperature, photoperiod, periods of drought or rain, food availability, reproductive mode and others (BASSI, 2016; PRADO, 2006).

The factors that make up the male reproductive cycle are firstly the acquisition of energy, followed by spermatogenesis, the production of secondary sexual characteristics, the search for copulation, dance-fighting, courtship and copulation (ZACARIOTTI, 2008).

2.3.1 Energy purchase

For both sexes, reproduction is costly, so it is necessary to acquire energy to complete the reproductive cycle. Snakes are still considered capital breeders, i.e. they don't reproduce until they have stockpiled the necessary amount of energy, so there is a separation of time for energy acquisition and the reproductive period (SUEIRO, 2013).

Males tend to store abdominal fat before gametogenesis, during the summer, which is mainly provided by food. In addition, there is a significant increase in the relative mass of the kidneys and the concentration of renal lipids, so the liposomatic, hepatosomatic and renalsomatic indices are accurate parameters for the mobilisation of energy substrates for both males and females (SUEIRO, 2013; PIZZATO, 2006a).

Depending on the need, such as the search for females and combat dances, energy is consumed and reaches a minimum at the end of the reproductive season (ZACARIOTTI, 2008). Energy costs are divided into two categories, linked to survival and fertility (SUEIRO, 2013).

2.3.2 Hormonal cycles

Few studies have described the relationship between reproductive behaviour, spermatogenesis and testosterone, but reproductive activity in reptiles, as in mammals, is controlled by the neuroendocrine system, with the hypothalamus releasing GnRH in response to environmental stimuli such as photoperiod, precisely because of the high demand for food and temperature. As a result, the anterior pituitary gland releases FSH-like hormones, which are only found in snakes and lizards, stimulating spermatogenesis (MATAYOSHI, 2011).

The amount of testosterone may be increased during the animals' reproductive and non-reproductive periods, thus showing that courtship and copulation are not dependent on an increase in testosterone levels (ALMEIDA-SANTOS, 2004). SALOMÃO and ALMEIDA-SANTOS

(2002) reported that in some species such as rattlesnakes, during reproductive behaviour there is an increase in testosterone, due to the basophilic precursors found in the adenohypophysis. During late summer and autumn, spermiogenesis takes place, but it is in autumn that spermatogenesis peaks, while in winter there is a phase of inactivity and testicular regression, which results in a lower level of testosterone (BARROS, 2012; ZACARIOTTI, 2010).

Two cycles are described in snakes: pre-nuptial and post-nuptial. The former is when the production of gametes precedes or coincides with the mating season, while in the latter the production of gametes occurs after the mating season, so the males need to store the sperm in the vas deferens, increasing its diameter, presenting copulation in the spring and testicular mass in the autumn (ALMEIDA-SANTOS, 2005; MOZAFARI, 2012; SILVA, 2015). BASSI (2016) described two other types of cycles: the mixed cycle, in which there is an increase in sperm production at the end of spring and an interruption during winter, and the acyclic cycle, in which production is constant throughout the year.

Currently, a new classification has been described by MATHIES (2011), dividing the cycles into individual levels, further separated into discontinuous cyclic, continuous cyclic and acyclic, and population levels. The discontinuous cycle is when the gonads completely retract in a given season, while the continuous cycle is when there is a reduction in gamete production and the acyclic cycle is when gamete production continues. Population can be synchronous or aseasonal, which shows synchrony or non-synchrony between individuals respectively.

1.2.1. Spermatogenesis and sperm morphology

For snakes, spermatogenesis is divided into five stages, the first of which has seminiferous tubules with a large number of spermatogonia and primary spermatocytes, compared to secondary spermatocytes and spermatids. In the second stage, the first sperm begin to appear, followed by the third stage with a large number of sperm in the seminiferous tubules, with a reduction in secondary spermatocytes and spermatids. The fourth stage sees a reduction in sperm and an increase in the number of spermatogonia and primary spermatocytes, while the fifth and final stage sees the presence of layers of spermatogonia and primary spermatocytes and the absence of sperm (ZACARIOTTI, 2004).

The sperm morphology of snakes described by ZACARIOTTI (2010) is a tapered sperm, with a cone-shaped acrosome and an elongated head. The intermediate part is quite long and is only attributed to snakes. This part contains the dense bodies, a possible mitochondrial transformation and the presence of proximal and distal centrioles, unlike mammals which only have one (Figure 12).

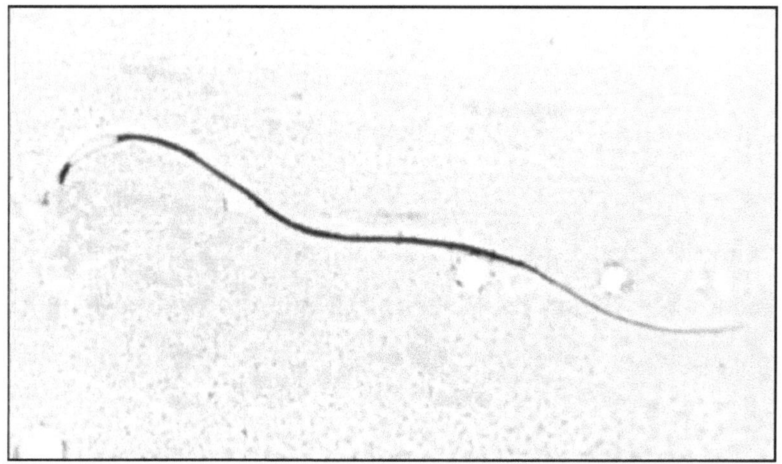

Figure 8: Normal morphology of rattlesnake (Crotalus durissus terrificus) sperm stained using simple acrosome staining (ZACARIOTTI, 2004).

1.2.2. Secondary sexual characteristics

Found in males concomitantly with gametogenesis. Snakes have a region of the kidneys called the SSR, consisting of regions of the distal convoluted tubule, collecting duct and ureter, which are stimulated in adults by high concentrations of steroid hormones such as testosterone in the bloodstream, producing granules of eosinophilic secretion and with the function of secreting substances for the maintenance of viable sperm during autumn (ZACARIOTTI, 2004; ALMEIDA-SANTOS, 2014; SUEIRO, 2013).

2.3.5 Dance combat

It's a male ritual during the mating season, characterised by non-aggressive bodily movements, through pushing, pinning or entangling the opponent, demonstrating their strength, but which can lead to the other individual's death, with the winner having priority over the female.

It occurs in different families, but mainly in those that are constrictors and/or poison their prey (PIZZATO, 2006b; SAWAYA, 2008; PIZZATO, 2006a).

Four combat patterns are found, in colubrids the males intertwine almost the entire body, with their heads close to and slightly above the ground, while elapids intertwine the entire body and the heads are parallel to the ground.

Mambas raise the anterior part of the trunk and intertwine, the heads are held vertically and the tails can be found intertwined or free. In viperids and crotalids, the trunk is elevated and loosely intertwined, with the heads also vertical and orientated face to face or in the same direction (Figure 13). An intermediate pattern is described for E. crassus, where a third of its body is elevated, remaining intertwined on the ground and strongly constricting each other (PIZZATO, 2006a).

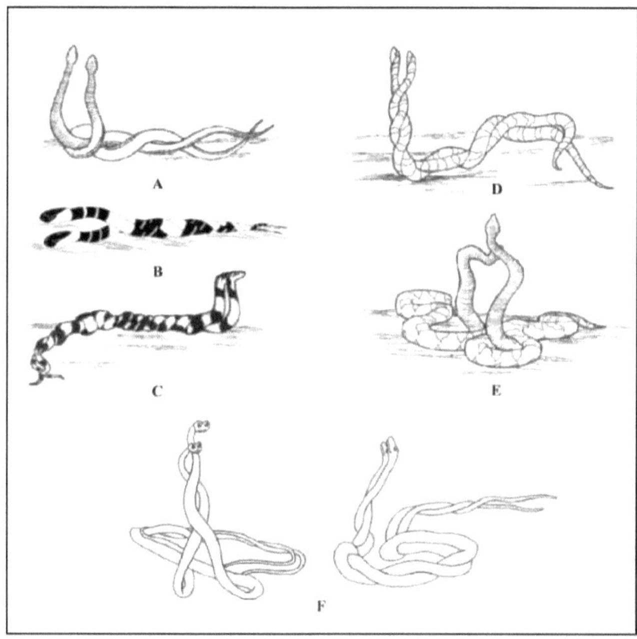

Figure 9: Characteristic postures during ritual combat. *Colubridae* Family - *Drymarchon corais* (A); *Elapidae Family - Micrutus frontalis* (B); Elapidae Family - *Bungarus fasciatus* (C); *Elapidae Family - Ophiophagus hannah* (D); *Viperidae Family - Crotalus durissus* (E); *Colubridae Family - Chironius bicarinatus* (F) (PIZZATO, 2006).

2.3.6. Cutting and copulation

As they are solitary animals, males tend to seek out females in the breeding season, using pherormones left by the female in the environment.

Courtship takes place in three phases, the first is tactile pursuit in which the male recognises and locates the female by chemical clues, the second is characterised by the alignment of the male on the female's back, in the Pythonidae the males can bite the female's body and in the Boidae the females are stimulated by spurs. The third phase is copulation itself, in which the tails of both animals intertwine and the female opens her cloaca for the hemipenis to penetrate (ZACARIOTTI, 2010; PIZZATO, 2006a).

Another reproductive strategy of snakes is the so-called multiple copulation, in which the female mates with several males in order to generate genetic variability. Inside the female's body, the best spermatozoa are also selected (PIZZATO, 2006a).

2.3.7. Sperm storage

Some snake species, both males and females, need a strategy for storing sperm, which varies from a few months to years, mainly because the time of spermatogenesis does not coincide with vitellogenesis (ZACARIOTTI, 2008; BARROS, 2012).

In males, sperm is stored in the distal part of the vas deferens and in females it is stored in the oviduct, by the formation of receptacles or storage tubules after copulation or in crypts in folds of the vaginal mucosa. To ensure that sperm survive for so long, new studies are being carried out, but there are indications that peptidases may be involved. This ability occurs mainly for the synchronisation of cycles (BASSI, 2016; ALMEIDA-SANTOS, 2005).

BASSI (2016) concluded in his study that SSR is rich in neutral carbohydrates and portions of peptide chains, so when they join with semen they serve as a source of energy for sperm survival and maintenance, especially when stored in the female oviduct.

2.4. Reproductive biotechnology

2.4.1. Semen collection

ZACARIOTTI (2010) mentioned in his article that the first semen collection in snakes took place in 1960, by compressing the final third of the animal's body, but contamination by faeces and urate was frequent. Continuing the experiment in 1980, he collected semen by ventrally massaging the final third of the animal's body, but with the aid of a syringe he collected the semen directly from the cloaca, minimising faecal contamination.

Continuing his studies, in 1989 he collected semen using an electroejaculator with subsequent digital massage, also in the ventral region, but just like the first, contamination was common. Another method found in the literature is semen collection by removing the animal's vas deferens after euthanasia, but this is less indicated (MOZAFARI, 2012; SILVA, 2017; ZACARIOTTI, 2010).

ZACARIOTTI (2004 and 2007) made a change to the technique described above, using a 1% lidocaine anaesthetic solution and ventral massage. The dose of lidocaine used was 15 mg/kg, diluted to a total volume of 1 mL of physiological solution. After this, the solution was fractionated into four injection sites anterior to the cloaca and applied to the subcutaneous tissue, thereby relaxing it and giving direct access to the genital papilla for collection using a 1 mL syringe without a needle. The species used in this study was *Crotalus durissus terrificus.*

With the efficacy of using local anaesthetics, studies with other species have been described, such as SILVA (2014), who assessed the sperm count of the *bothrops insularis*. The results showed little variation in sperm vigour and volume during the seasons, lower motility during the summer and a different concentration during the winter.

2.4.2. Macroscopic and microscopic evaluation

In order to know the normal parameters of the species and assess the male's reproductive potential, it is necessary to carry out a spermogram, but there are still few reports on snakes (ZACARIOTTI, 2010).

As snake semen is highly concentrated, a pre-dilution is recommended for subsequent analysis, and these dilutions can be around 1:500 as described by ZACARIOTTI (2007) or 1:1000 as shown in the study by SILVA (2014). Cell culture media are the most suitable for dilution, such as M199, Hanrís F10, PBS and TL Hepes solution. As snakes are ectodermic animals, there is no need to use heating plates; the ideal temperature for them is between 25 and 27°C (ZACARIOTTI, 2010).

Semen is analysed macroscopically for volume, density, colour and odour, and microscopically for turbidity, motility, vigour, sperm concentration and sperm pathologies. There is also a division into immediate tests (carried out immediately after collection) and mediate tests (carried out after collection, but analysed later), so the immediate tests are sperm volume, colour, density, odour, motility and vigour, and the mediate tests are sperm concentration and pathologies (PAPA, 2014).

ALMEIDA-SANTOS (2014) and ZACARIOTTI (2004) describe the

following characteristics of snakes:

-Volume   : 0.5 to 10 μL (estimated using a micropipette);

-Appearance : Watery to milky;

-Colour : Greyish white to milky;

-Odor   : *suis generis;*

-Turbulence : 0 to 5;

-Motility   : 50 to 70 per cent;

-Vigour : 4 to 5;

2.4.3   Cryopreservation

The cryopreservation of snake semen is still little studied, so few techniques are described in the literature. The most commonly used diluents are milk, coconut water, Ham's F10 and test-gema (ZACARIOTTI, 2008; SALVADOR, 2016). SAMOUR (2004) says that glycerol is toxic to the sperm of the species in question, but the study by ZACARIOTTI (2006) proved that it is not.

On the contrary, it managed to maintain a motility of 70 per cent immediately after thawing, using test-gema and 8 per cent glycerol as diluent.

Techniques for cryopreserving semen have been described since 1980, and over the years the techniques have been modified and improved. In the first studies, McCoy's modified cell culture medium was used as the diluent for refrigeration and the sperm motility of the viable sample was maintained up to 96 hours after the procedure. The same author also froze the sperm with a commercial diluent and obtained 30% motility after thawing

(ZACARIOTTI, 2010).

In 2007, FAHRING in his experiment managed to leave the semen of the corn snake (Pantherophis guttatus) with sperm motility greater than 50 % for 48 hours, using test-yolk and cooling the sample to 4°C. In the same year, MATTSON used the same species, but with a different protocol, in which the semen was diluted in TL herpes solution to assess sperm concentration and managed to maintain motility between 70 and 95 per cent for three days at a refrigeration temperature of 4 to 10°C.

In his experiment, ZACARIOTTI (2008) used test-gema and Lake's diluent as diluents, with 4 different freezing protocols: the first consisted of dripping the sample into liquid nitrogen (pellet), the second used a specific container for freezing, the 5100 Cryo 1° and protocol three and four the samples were placed in a freezing machine with two different protocols. Three different protocols were used for defrosting, after 10 minutes of waiting.

2.4.4 Artificial insemination

For the artificial insemination of snakes, the techniques developed use fresh or refrigerated semen. There are no reports of frozen semen being deposited in the oviducts of females, so localising this organ in the cloaca is important. To do this, probes are used, which can be flexible or rigid, the ideal size for the female, and a syringe containing the semen is attached to the end of the probe. The moment when the semen is deposited has not yet been well described, but some authors have used the animal's natural copulation period (ZACARIOTTI, 2010; ZACARIOTTI, 2008).

Even in the studies that were successful in insemination, the number of offspring was reduced when compared to natural copulation. The reproduction of these animals is hampered mainly by the lack of literature on reptile physiology (ZACARIOTTI, 2010; ZACARIOTTI, 2008).

CHAPTER 3

METHODOLOGY

3.1. Animals

Firstly, in order to carry out the project, it was submitted to the Ethics Committee of the Faculdades Integradas de Ourinhos (FIO) in March 2017, under process 2017/009, and the approval protocol was 009/2017.

Seven (100%) male snakes were evaluated, four belonging to the Epicrates crassus species (57.15%) (Figure 14A), two to the Python regius species (28.57%) (Figure 14B) and one to the Crotalus durissus terrificus species (14.28%) (Figure 14C). All the animals belong to the IPEVS, located in the city of Cornélio Procópio - PR. For each animal, a general assessment form was drawn up containing the animal's age, data on feeding, enclosure structure and cloacal rostral length, and on another specific form for each animal, data was recorded regarding the clinical examination, containing behaviour, nutritional status, water intake, food intake, weight, hydration level, appearance of the skin and appendages, data on palpation, muscle tone, urination and defecation (Table 6A and 6B).

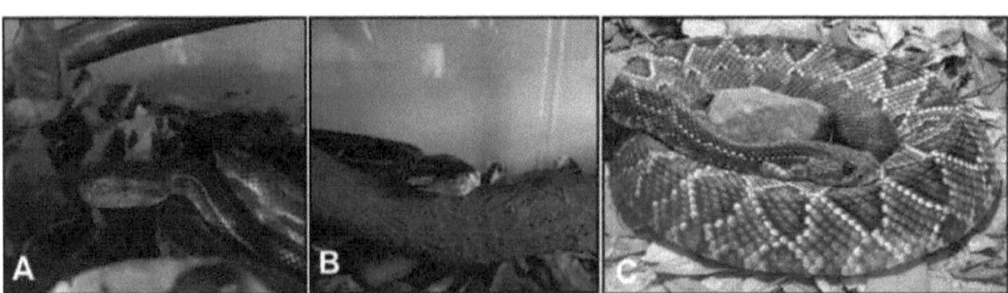

Figure 10: Animals used in the experiment. Salamanta (Epicrates crassus) (A); Ball python (Python regius) (B); Rattlesnake (Crotalus durissus terrificus) (C) (Source: Personal archive).

3.2 Semen collection

The semen was collected using the method described by MENGDEN et al. (1980), in which a digital massage was carried out on the ventral region of the final third of the animal and the semen was collected directly into the cloaca using a 1mL syringe, in order to avoid contamination of the biological material with faeces and urine that could be present in the area.

Firstly, for collection, the animals were physically restrained in a plastic tube and placed in a supine position. Ventral massages were then carried out for 20 minutes to eject the semen (Figures 15A and 15B), after which it was collected using a 1 mL syringe and then placed on a glass slide or imprinted in the region of the cloaca (Figures 16A and 16B) and overlaid with a coverslip for evaluation under optical microscopy at 40x magnification.

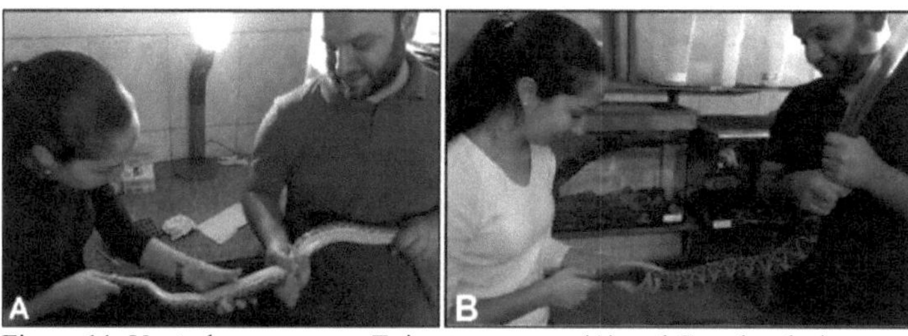

Figure 11: Ventral massages on Epicrates crassus (A) and Crotalus durissus terrificus (B) (Source: Personal archive).

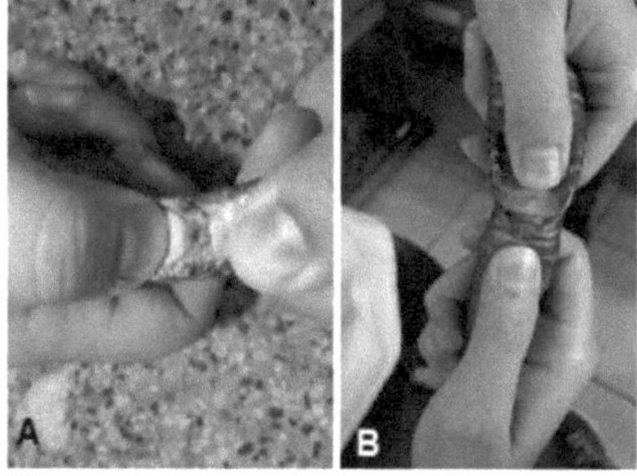

Figure 12: Cloaca region in Epicrates crassus (A) and Crotalus durissus terrificus (B) (Source: Personal archive).

In all, the experiment consisted of four semen collections for the E. crassus snakes, while two collections were made for the P. regiuse C. durissus. The interval between the first three collections was approximately one month and between the third and fourth collection was only 48 hours.

Table 4a: Results obtained after the general assessment and anamnesis of the animals.

Species	*E. crassus* (1)	*E. crassus* (2)	*E. crassus* (3)	*S. crassus* (4)
GENERAL EVALUATION				
Age	20 years	7 years	7 years	7 years
Food	Mice	Mice	Mice	Mice
Venue structure	Plastic box with corrugated cardboard	Plastic box with corrugated cardboard	Substrate with leaves (exposure)	Plastic box with corrugated cardboard
CRC	89 cm	83 cm	89 cm	88 cm
CLINICAL EXAMINATION				
Behaviour	Docile	Docile	Docile	Docile
Nutritional status	Normal	Normal	Normal	Normal
Water intake	*Ad libitum*	*Ad libitum*	*Ad libitum*	*Ad libitum*
Food intake	Normal	Normal	Normal	Normal
Weight	894 gr	787 gr	738 gr	787 gr
Moisturising	Hydrated	Hydrated	Hydrated	Hydrated
Skin and appendages	Scar	Normal	Normal	Normal
Palpation	No volume increase	No volume increase	No volume increase	No volume increase
Muscle tone	Normal	Normal	Normal	Normal
Urination and defecation	Normal	Normal	Normal	Normal

Chart 4b: Results obtained after the general assessment and anamnesis of the animals.

Species	*P. regius* (5)	*P. regius* (6)	*C. durissus* (7)
GENERAL EVALUATION			
Age	20 years	8 years	Free life
Food	Mice	Mice	Mice
Venue structure	Substrate with leaves (exposure)	Substrate with leaves	Plastic box with corrugated cardboard
CRC	1.17 cm	1.03 cm	96 cm
CLINICAL EXAMINATION			
Behaviour	Docile	Docile	Docile
Nutritional status	Normal	Normal	Normal
Water intake	*Ad li bitu m*	*Ad libitum*	*Ad libitum*
Food intake	Normal	Normal	Normal

Weight	2,149kg	2,146kg	1,118kg
Moisturising	Hydrated	Hydrated	Hydrated
Skin and appendages	Normal	Normal	Normal
Palpation	No volume increase	No volume increase	No volume increase
Muscle tone	Normal	Normal	Normal
Urination and defecation	Normal	Normal	Normal

CHAPTER 4

RESULTS AND DISCUSSION

The collection method used in this study was ventral massaging of the animal, with physical restraint, which is considered a safe method for both the animal and the handler. In addition, collection using a syringe minimises contamination by urate and faeces in the semen, as described by MENGDEN (1980), ZACARIOTTI (2004 and 2007) and SILVA (2014). Other methods have been described, such as compressing the final third of the animal's body and using an electroejaculator, but in both cases contamination of the sample was common (FITCH, 1960; QUINN, 1989). There have also been studies that have collected semen after euthanising the animal, such as MOZAFARI (2012) and TOURMENTE (2006).The variation in results, which are described in Table 7, can be attributed to the characteristics of the species of animal analysed, such as habitat use, predation techniques and feeding habits.

Table 5: Results obtained after stimulating the male for sperm collection.

	1° harvest	2° harvest	3° harvest	4° harvest
E. crassus (1)	Spermatozoa -from property	Immobile sperm	No sperm	No sperm
E. crassus (2)	Without sperm	No sperm	No sperm	No sperm
E. crassus (3)	Mucus, no sperm -des	No sperm	No sperm	No sperm
E. crassus (4)	Without sperm	Immobile sperm	No sperm	No sperm
P. regius (5)	Not collected	Not collected	Immobile sperm	No sperm

P. regius (6)	Not collected	Not collected	Immobile sperm	No sperm
C. durissus (7)	Not collected	Not collected	Viable sperm	No sperm

In his study, JAYNE (1982) presents adaptive differences between the musculature of arboreal, terrestrial and aquatic snakes. However, according to PIZZATTO (2009), E. crassus have terrestrial habits, mainly due to their robust body shape. This can also be said of P. regius and C. durissus (GRAF, 2011; ALMEIDA-SANTOS, 2005).

Both E. crassus and P. regius are animals with aglyphic dentition, which kill their prey by constriction, i.e. by asphyxiation or circulatory arrest. Unlike these two species, C. durissus are animals with solenoglyphic dentition, i.e. they have fangs for venom inoculation and kill their prey by envenomation, making it a venomous species.

Constrictor snakes have significant morphological differences when compared to venomous snakes. As well as having a greater number of vertebrae, which gives them greater flexibility, they also have a greater number of short axial muscle segments, capable of producing a greater force of contraction (JAYNE, 1982).

The hypothesis raised here is based on the difficulty encountered in collecting semen using the ventral massage technique in the constrictor snakes used in this study, which could be attributed to the force of muscle contraction exerted by the specimens during collection, which would obviously result in the massage not being effective in guiding the sperm towards the genital papilla. This hypothesis could be based on the studies of JAYNE (1982), who states that shorter muscle segments could increase the force of contraction, as a greater number of complete muscle segments could fit into a given body length.

The time taken for the ventral massages did not exceed the 20 minutes proposed in the study's methodology, but there was variation between the snakes, whether they were of the same species or not. Some did not ejaculate during these periods and others, such as C. durissus, ejaculated after 15 minutes of massage.

In C. durissus, the only animal in which viable sperm was collected, it can be observed:

- Volume: not estimated
- Swirling: 4
- Motility (%): 90
- Vigour: 5

The other parameters were not assessed due to the small volume of samples taken. Thus, the results obtained for turbulence and vigour corroborate the reference values for the species described in the literature, while motility is above normal values.

CHAPTER 5

CONCLUSION

Taking into account what was observed, we can conclude that the method of collecting sperm by ventral massage using a syringe, described by MENGDEN (1980), proved to be satisfactory for Crotalus durissus terrificus, while for Python regius and Epicrates crassus the efficiency was low, resulting in the collection of immobile sperm. This could be explained by the fact that the latter two animals are constrictors and thus have more developed muscles than the former. As a result, further studies should be carried out with both species.

REFERENCES

ALMEIDA-SANTOS, Selma Maria. **Reproductive Models in Snakes: Sperm Storage in** Crotalus durissus **and** Bothrops jararaca **(Serpentes:** Viperidae**).** 2005. 206 f. Dissertation (Doctorate) - Faculty of Veterinary Medicine and Zootechny, University of São Paulo, São Paulo, 2005.

ALMEIDA, F. S.; CONTE, A. V.; SANT' ANNA, S. S.; FERNANDES, W.; GREGO, K. F. Topographic Localisation and Ultrasound Imaging of the Internal Organs of the Jararaca (Bothrops jararaca, Serpentes, Viperidae). In: ABRAVAS Congress. Campos do Jordão. Proceedings of **the XIII ABRAVAS Congress,** p. 67-70, 2010.

ALMEIDA-SANTOS, Selma Maria. et al. Reproductive Biology of Snakes: Recommendations for Data Collection and Analysis. **Herpetologia Brasileira,** v.3, n. 1, p. 14 - 24, mar, 2014.

ANDRADE, A.; PINTO, SC.; OLIVEIRA, RS. **Laboratory animals**: breeding and experimentation[online]. Rio de Janeiro: Editora FIOCRUZ, 2002. 388 p. ISBN: 85-7541-015-6. <http://books.scielo.org>.

BARROS, Verônica Alberto; SUEIRO, Letícia Ruiz; ALMEIDA-SANTOS, Selma Maria. Reproductive Biology of the Neotropical Rattlesnake Crotalus durissus from Northeastern Brazil: a Test of Phylogenetic Conservatism of Reproductive Patterns. **Herpetological journal**, v. 22, p. 97-104, 2012.

BASSI, Erick Augusto. **The Influence of Climatic Variations on the Reproductive Cycle of True Corals** Micrurus corallinus **and *Micrurus frontalis*.** 2016. 111 f. Master's Degree - Institute of Biosciences, Letters and Exact Sciences, São Paulo State University, São José do Rio Preto, 2016.

CARVALHO, Celso Morato; ALENCAR, Inês Cristina de Souza; VILAR, Jeane Carvalho. Snakes of the Manaus Region, Central Amazonia, Brazil. **General and Experimental Biology**, v. 7, n. 2, p. 41-59, 2007.

CHARLES, Henrique Abrahão. **Predatory Behaviour of Snakes (*Boidae*) of Different Habits and Growth Biometry and Ecdysis of *Eunectes murinus* Linnaeus, 1758 in the Laboratory.** 2007. 82 f. Dissertation (Master's Degree) - Institute of Biology, Federal Rural University of Rio de Janeiro, Seropédica, 2007.

COSTA, Henrique Caldeira; MOURA, Mário Ribeiro; FEIO, Renato Alves. **Snakes of Viçosa and Region (Minas Gerais)**. Belo Horizonte: FAPEMIG, Viçosa: UFV, 2008. 28.

FAHRIG, B. M.; MITCHELL, M. A.; EILTS, B. E.; PACCAMONTI, D. L. Characterisation and cooled storage of semen from corn snakes (Elaphe guttata). **J Zoo Wild Med**, v.38, p.7-12, 2007.

FITCH, H. S. Criteria for determining sex and breeding maturity in snakes. **Herpetology**, v.16, p.49-51, 1960.

FRAGA, Rafael. et al. **Guide to Snakes of the Manaus Region - Central Amazonia.** Manaus: Inpa, 2013. 303.

GARCIA, Viviane Campos. **Ultrasonographic Evaluations of the Reproductive Cycles of Neotropical Boidae Snakes.** 2012. Dissertation (Master's Degree) - Faculty of Veterinary Medicine and Zootechny, University of São Paulo, São Paulo, 2012.

GARCIA, Viviane Campos. et al. Ultrasonographic Evaluation of the Reproductive Apparatus in Viviparous Snakes of the Boidae Family. **Pesq. Vet. Bras.**, v. 35, n. 3, p. 311-318, mar, 2015.

GRAF, A. "Python regius" (On-line), **Animal Diversity Web**, Michigan, 2011. Available at : <http://animaldiversity.org/accounts/Python_regius/>. Accessed on: 11 October 2017.

GREGO, Kathleen Fernandes; ALBUQUERQUE, Luciana Rameh; KOLESNIKOVAS, Cristiane Kiyomii Miyaji. Squamata (Snakes). InCUBAS, Zalmir Silvino; SILVA, Jean Carlos Ramos; CATÃO-DIAS, José Luiz. **Treatise on Wild Animals**. São Paulo: Roca, 2014. p.186-218.

IRIZARRY, Kristopher; RUTLLANT, Josep. Leveraging Comparative Genomics to Identify and Functionally Characterise Genes Associated with Sperm Phenotypes in *Python bivittatus* (Burmese Python). **Genetics Research International**, p. 1-16, 2016.

JANEIRO-CINQUINI, Thélia. Annual Variation in the Reproductive System of Female Bothrops jararaca (Serpentes: Viperidae). **Sér. Zool.**, v. 94, n. 3, p. 325-328, sep, 2004.

JAYNE, B. C. Comparative Morphology of the Semispinalis-Spinalis Muscles of Snakes and Correlations with Locomotion and Constriction. **Journal of Morphology**. 1982.

MATAYOSHI, Priscilla Mitie. **Ultrasonographic and Morphophysiological Characterisation of the Reproductive System of Males and Females of *Crotalus durissus terrificus*.** 2011. 108 f. Dissertation (Master's) - Faculty of Veterinary Medicine and Zootechnics, Universidade Estadual Paulista, Botucatu, 2011.

MATAYOSHI, Priscilla Mitie. et al. Ultrasound evaluation of the coelomatic cavity of snakes. **Vet. e Zootec.**, v. 19, n. 4, p. 448459, 2012.

MATHIES, T. Reproductive Cycles of Tropical Snake. In: ALDRIDGE, R.

D.; SEVER, D. M. **Reproductive Biology and Philogeny of Snake**. Enfield: Science Publishers, p. 511-550, 2011.

MATTSON, K. J.; VRIES, A. D, MCGUIRE, S. M.; KREBS, J.; LOUIS, E. E.; LOSKUTOFF, N. M. Successful artificial insemination in the corn snake (Elaphe gutatta), using fresh and cooled semen. **Zoo Biol**, v.26, p.363-369, 2007.

MENGDEN, A. G.; PLATZ, G. C.; HUBBARD, R.; QUINN, H. Semen collection, freezing and artificial insemination in snakes. In: Murphy

JB. Reproductive biology and diseases of captive reptiles. Lawrence, KS: **The Society for the study of Amphibians and Reptiles,** p.71- 78, 1980.

MOZAFARI, Sayedeh Zahra; SHIRAVI, Abdolhossein; TODEHDEHGHAN, Fatemeh. Evaluation of Reproductive Parameters of Vas Deferens Sperms in Caucasian Snake (Gloydius halys caucasicus). **Veterinary Research Forum**, v. 3, n. 2, p. 119123, 2012.

PASSOS, Paulo; FERNANDES, Ronaldo. Revision of the Epicrates cenchria Complex (Serpentes: Boidae). **Herpetological Monographs**, n. 22, p. 1-30, 2008.

PAPA, Frederico Ozanam. et al. **Manual of Andrology and Equine Semen Handling**. 2014.

PIZZATTO, Ligia; ALMEIDA-SANTOS, Selma Maria; MARQUES,

Otávio Augusto Vuolo. **Reproductive biology of Brazilian snakes**. Herpetology in Brazil. 2006 (a).

PIZZATTO, Ligia; MANFIO, Rafael Haddad; ALMEIDA-SANTOS, Selma Maria. Male-male ritualised combat in the Brazilian rainbow boa, Epicrates cenchria crassus. **Herpetological Bulletin**, n.95, p. 16 - 20,2006 (b).

PIZZATTO, L.; MARQUES, O. A. V; FACURE, K. Food habits of Brazilian boid snakes: overview and new data, with special reference

to Corallus hortulanus. **Amphibia-Reptilia**, v. 30, n. 4, p. 533-544, 2009.

PRADO, Lígia Pizzatto. **Ecomorphology and Reproductive Strategies in** Boidae **(Snakes), with Emphasis on Neotropical Species.** 162 f. Doctoral dissertation - Institute of Biology, State University of Campinas, Campinas, 2006.

QUINN, H.; BLASEDEL, T.; PLATZ, C. C. Successful artificial insemination in the checked garter snake. **Int Zoo Yb**, v.28, p.177- 183, 1989.

SALOMÃO, M. G. & ALMEIDA-SANTOS, S.M. The reproductive cycle in male neotropical rattlesnakes (Crotalus durissus terrificus). In: SCHUETT, G.W.; HOGGREN, M.; DOUGLAS, M.E. & GREENE, H.W. (eds.) **Biology of the Vipers**. Indiana: Carmel, p.507-514, 2002.

SALVADOR, Pablo Simón; TRILLO, Agustin Álvarez; MARCORRO, Gisela Fuentes. Hypoosmotic Shock in Cascabel Viper Sperm. **Revista Iberoamericana de Ciencias**, v. 3, n. 3, p. 52-57, 2016.

SAMOUR, J. H. Semen Collection, Spermatozoa Cryopreservation, and Artificial Insemination in Nondomestic Birds. **Journal of Avian Medicine and Surgery**, v. 18, n. 4, p. 219-223, 2004.

SAWAYA, Ricardo Jannini; MARQUES, Otávio Augusto Vuolo; MARTINS, Marcio. Composition and Natural History of the Snakes of

Cerrado of Itirapina, São Paulo, Southeastern Brazil. **Biota Neotrop**, v. 8, n. 2, p. 127-149, Apr/Jun, 2008.

SCARTOZZONI, Rodrigo Roveri; MOLINA, Flávio de Barros. Feeding Behaviour of Boa constrictor, Epicrates cenchria and Corallus hortulanus (Serpentes: Boidae) in Captivity. **Revista de Etologia**, v. 6, n. 1, p. 25-31, 2004.

SILVA, Kalena Barros. **Evaluation of the Spermogram of Bothrops insularis, (Snakes: Viperidae) Kept in Captivity**. 53 f. 2014. Dissertation (Master's Degree) - Faculty of Veterinary Medicine and Zootechny, University of São Paulo, São Paulo, 2014.

SILVA, Karina Maria Pereira. **Reproductive Biology of the Amazonian Jararaca,** Bothrops atrox **(Serpent:** Viperidae**)**. 82 f. 2015. Dissertation (Master's Degree) - Faculty of Veterinary Medicine and Zootechny, University of São Paulo, São Paulo, 2015.

SILVA, A. C. et al. Evaluation of sperm quality of Erythrolamprus poecilogyrus sublineatus (Cope, 1860) (Serpentes, Dipsadidae). **Braz. J.**

Biol., Aug, 2017.

SUEIRO, Letícia Ruiz. **Reproductive Costs in** Crotalus durissus **(Serpentes, Viperidae) from the State of São Paulo, Brazil**. 2013. 102 f. Doctoral dissertation - Faculty of Veterinary Medicine and Zootechny, University of São Paulo, São Paulo, 2013.

TOURMENTE, M.; CARDOZO, G.; GUIDOBALDI, H.; GIOJALAS, L.; BERTONA, M.; CHIARAVIGLIO, M. The ultrastructure of the spermatozoa of Boa constrictor occidentalis, with considerations on its mating system and sperm competition theories. **Acta Zool**, v.87, p.25-32, 2006.

ZACARIOTTI, Rogério Loesch. **Longitudinal study of the spermogram and serum testosterone levels of rattlesnakes (Crotalus durissus terrificus, Laurenti, 1768) from the wild in the state of São Paulo**. 2004. 80 f. Dissertation (Master's Degree) - Faculty of Veterinary Medicine and Zootechny, University of São Paulo, São Paulo, 2004.

ZACARIOTTI, Rogério Loesch; DURRANT, Barbara. The Bud Heller Conservation Fellowship for 2005: Assisted Reproduction in Snakes. **Conservation and Research for Endangered Species**, 2006.

ZACARIOTTI, Rogério Loesch. Assisted Reproduction in Reptiles. **Fowler Group**, chap. 12, Apr, 2007.

ZACARIOTTI, Rogério Loesch. **Reproductive evaluation and freezing of**

snake semen. 2008. 98 f. Doctoral dissertation - Faculty of Veterinary Medicine and Zootechny, University of São Paulo, São Paulo, 2008.

ZACARIOTTI, R.L; GUIMARÃES, M.A.B.V.Applications of biotechnology in snake reproduction. **Brazilian Journal of Animal Reproduction**. Belo Horizonte. v.34, n.2,p. 98 - 104 apr./jun. 2010.

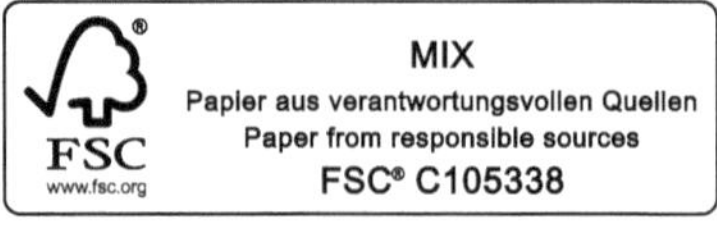

Printed by Books on Demand GmbH, Norderstedt / Germany